CN

A

EXAM PREPARATION
2018 - 2019

North Carolina State:
Skills Board Exam

CNA Skills Study Guide with all the 22 skills and checkpoints. For everybody who want to challenge and pass the NORTH CAROLINA STATE CNA SKILLS STATE BOARD EXAM without any prior experience.

THANK YOU FOR PURCHASING MY BOOK: PLEASE GIVE ME AN HONEST AFTER READING THE BOOK AND GOOD LUCK WITH CNA SKILLS STATE BOARDS EXAM

Disclaimer

Introduction

T

his book is customized for NORTH CAROLINA STATE CNA STUDENTS: To Prepare them tor the Skills portion of the State Boards Exam. The books Highlights all the checkpoints examiners look for in the Skills performance part of the exam. It also gives you the step by step guide on performing each skills in the NORTH CAROLINA STATE BOARDS EXAM. The hidden secrets and everything the student needs to know. It should be noted the word PATIENT/ RESIDENT IS USED INTERCHANGEABLY

Table of Contents

WHO IS A CNA?

A

 Certified Nursing Assistant (CNA) is an important member of the healthcare team. They are primarily involved in offering direct care to the patients. They also assist members of the healthcare chain of command including the nurses, doctors. They spend most time with the patients than any other member of the healthcare team. A CNA works under the supervision of a nurse to deliver adequate care to the patient. Their job demands long working hours and a lot of responsibilities. Their

job description is to majorly help patients with Activities of the Daily Living (ADL) even though their job is not limited to that. A CNA can work in various places like hospitals, adult care facilities, personal homes, nursing homes etc. In a hospital setting, the usual duties of a CNA are listed below

• Taking and making a record of vitals e.g. blood pressure, blood sugar level, Pulse, Respiration etc.

• Patient observation and reporting the observation to the necessary professional

• Help in cleaning the patient and the ambulating the patient. They also bathe, dress and feed their patients and make the patient's bed.

• CNA helps in changing the patient's position

These are the general duties of a CNA. There are many illnesses that could require the assistant of a CNA For more illustration on what a CNA does, let us examine a patient with stroke for example. A patient with stroke most likely is not able to talk or walk. They also cannot perform some activities of daily living e.g. dress him/herself, range of motion, ambulation, moving from one position to another, brushing, feeding etc. The CNA assists the patients in performing these activities.

Some of the strengths that are required of a CNA includes: team work, empathy, a good sense of humor, ability to manage time, adaptability, communication skills and a good knowledge of patients in the facility. It is important that a good CNA has the necessary skill set to be able to carry out these duties appropriately.

To become a qualified CNA, you have to pass the Certified Nursing Assistant Examination. This examination is divided into two segments which are the clinical skills test and the written examination. This ebook is focused on the clinical skill test which is the practical aspect of the examination. This book contains step by step explanation on the clinical skills a CNA should possess. It has been designed to equip you with the adequate step by step information required to excel in this.

Chapter 1

The Clinical Skill Test

s said earlier, the NORTH CAROLINA clinical skills test Evaluates the CNA student ability to perform all the 22 Skills accurately and applying all the FIVE Principles of Care in each every Skill in the Exam Before you start your begin your CLINICAL Skills exam. There Examiner/Nurse will give you instructions to follow for the exam and including what to do if need to correct yourself. You will also be given time to familiarize yourself with the exam room and where locate all the supplies required for the exam. It also helps authenticate the ability of a future CNA to perform the responsibilities of a nursing assistant. Here are the FIVE principles of Care to review and understand. : **Infection control, Privacy, Safety, Dignity and communication/indirect care.**

• **Hand washing is the infection control.**

You need to make sure your hands are clean and free from germs before and after any procedure.

• **Privacy:**

This involves maintaining the privacy of the patient as you commence work. Did you close the door or the curtains?

• **Safety:**

You have to ensure you take necessary precautions when carrying out any procedure. The safety of your patients and even yourself is of importance. Did you lower the bed after completing the skill? Ensure the equipments are fully functional.

• Dignity:

Ensure you cover up part of the patient's body that you are not working on. Expose only areas that are involved in the skill.

• Indirect care:

This means actively talking to the resident or patient. You have to explain every process to them making sure your patient is really comfortable as you work. You could ask simple questions like: "Are you okay, Miss Suzie?" say your patient's name is Miss Suzie.

These five principles must be applied as you perform your skills. As much as it is important to know the 22 skills, you are going to be tested on Three random skills, one of which is recordable. Two nurses will be present to evaluate your performance throughout the five principles listed above. After the completion of the test, the nurses will record their observations into a computer. The nurse who is facilitating the test will give you basic rules on how to make corrections when testing. The Prometric's system determines the results based on the recorded results by the nurse during observation of your performance.

The nurse who is facilitating the test will provide basic rules on how to make connections while testing. I highly recommend that you familiarize yourself with the testing room and the places where all the supplies are located. The testing room will have a setup similar to a resident's room. The following personal care supplies will be found in the resident's bedside cabinet;

- 1st drawer contains toothbrush, toothpaste, Denture brush

- 2nd drawer contains basins, lotion and soap

• 3rd drawer contains bedpans, urinals, graduate

OPENING STATEMENT

As a CNA, promoting patient's right is a vital part of the job. Here is example of the Opening Statement.

Step 1 Knock Knock?

Step 2 Can i come in?

Step 3 Greet the resident by their name: "Good morning Ms Suzie"

Step 4 Introduce yourself and your title: "My name is Mary and i am your CNA for today"

Step 5 Tell the patient why you are in their room: "I came to mention the task you came to do"

Step 6 Ask if the time is good for them to do the skill: "Is this a good time?"

Step 7 Acknowledge the resident's call light: "I see your call light is within reach, (make sure the call light is indeed within the patient's hand to reach) I am going to wash my hands and close the curtain for privacy before we begin".

Step 8 Then leave the room and go wash your hands; If the this is the FIRST SKILL in the exam, you would need to wash your hands PHYSICALLY. Second and Third skill you can just pretend (Verbally say wash my hands) to wash your hands.

Step 9 Then close the curtain and return back to the resident's bed to begin your skill.

Step 10 Communicate everything with the patient while performing the skill; this is called INDIRECT CARE .

Step 11 Keep your eyes on the patient throughout your skill to to make sure you can read their facial expression incase your patient had a stroke and is unable to speak.

This serves as the opening statement.

NOTE: **Since the opening statement has been discussed here, it will not be repeated for each skill. Please take note of this and practice it.**

CLOSING STATEMENT

We are going to use our resident Ms Suzie as an example

    Step 1: Ms Suzie I am done

    Step 2: Is there anything else i can do for you before i leave

    Step 3: Would you like fresh cup of water, watch tv or read a magazine

    Step 4: Okay i see your call light is within reach(make sure you put it close to the resident's hand)

    Step 5: I am going to open the curtain for sunshine and wash my hands

    Step 6: If you need anything else please press the call light

.

e

Handwashing Skill

T

he two nurses will appraise your hand washing skill. One of them will observe hand washing at the beginning of the First skill while the other will observe at the end of the First skill.

Please note that there will be no instruction to wash your hands because you should know that hand washing is necessary. You are expected to wash your hands before you start the first skill, that is, after your opening statement. The first nurse will observe your hand washing skill at this stage. After the first skill has been done, it is essential that you wash your hands again. This time, the second nurse will be the observer.

For the next two skills, you are required to VERBALLY say "wash my hands, wash my hands, pat dry, and pat dry my hands". You are not expected to PHYSICALLY wash your hands if it is not your first skill.

HANDWASHING TECHNIQUES

The time required to wash your hands is 3minutes.

You can use the 6 paper towels method for this technique.

The steps include:

Step 1: Take the first paper towel, turn on the faucet and feel the temperature of the water while holding the paper towel. Ensure that the water is lukewarm before disposing the paper towel.

Step 2: Wet your hands without touching the inside of the sink

Step 3: Get a generous amount of soap on your hands, rub them together facing them down counting up to 20 seconds

Step 4: Wash between fingers three times

Step 5: Wash cuticles three times

Step 6: Wash underneath the nails three times

Step 7: Wash the inside of your hands by scrubbing with the top of your fingers

Step 8: Rub your wrist rigorously three times

Step 9: Grab the second paper towel and pat dry your hands from the finger tips gently towards the wrist, and dispose off the towel

Step 10: Grab the third paper towel and pat dry the same hand completely dry

Step 11: Grab the fourth paper towel and pat dry the other hand, gently repeating what you did with the previous hand

Step 12: Grab the fifth paper towel and pat dry the hand completely

Step 13: Grab the last paper towel and then turn off the water. Make sure you do not recontaminate the hand

e

Passive Range of Motion
(ROM) exercises to one shoulder

The time required for this skill is 4-5 minutes.

There are no supplies for this skill.

R

ange of motion exercise to One Shoulder tests on flexing and extending resident's shoulder by raising the arm all the way towards the head of the bed and all the way back to to the bed/mattress three times. The second exercise is to move the resident's Shoulder away from their body ABDUCTION towards the side and bringing the shoulder back ADDUCTION towards their body three times. Its important to exercise the right joint (SHOULDER) when you do ROM to One Shoulder. You are going to be tested on the CORRECT SIDE. Make sure you exercise the correct side. Meaning either the LEFT or the RIGHT SHOULDER Make sure to ask the resident if they feel pain or not and to also keep your eyes on their face to observe if they are in pain

Step 1 : Start your skill with your opening statement.

Step 2: Begin the exercise only one shoulder, make sure it is the correct side

Step 3: Hold the resident's arm and shoulder, raise it up FLEXION/towards the head of the bed and EXTENSION/lower it back to the mattress slowly and gently. Repeat this process three times

Step 4: Hold resident's shoulder and arm then move it away from their body outwards ABDUCTION/towards the side and bring back ADDUCTION/towards their body. Repeat this process three times.

Step 5: Make sure you communicate with the patient while performing the skill. Ask the patient about their comfort intermittently

Step 6: Make sure you keep your eyes on the patient's face. This is so you can see the expressions on the resident's face for example if he is in pain.

Step 7: Remember to support the patient's extremity while you work on the joint during the skill. This is to ensure they are protected.

Step 8: Close your skill by going over the closing statement

Step 9: Take into consideration patient's safety rights- Don't forget to lower the bed, Place the call light next to the patient's strong hand, Put the over bed tray beside the resident's bed and open the curtains

Step 10: Finally, ensure you wash your hands. Physically, if it is the first skill of the exam or verbally if it is the second or third skill

Chapter 4

e

Passive range of motion
(ROM) exercise to one elbow and wrist

The time duration for this skill is 4-5 minutes.

There are no supplies.

T

his skill involves providing range of motion exercise to a resident's ELBOW by making FLEXING/EXTENDING it. Next you are going to FLEX/HYPEREXTEND the WRIST. Because this is a test you are only required to repeat each exercise THREE TIMES The examiner will notify you in terms of which side of the patient you need to work on. LEFT/RIGHT side of the patient's elbow and wrist.

Ensure you look at the resident's face and maintain communication with the patient as you perform this skill.

    Step 1: Start your skill with your opening statement.

    Step 2: Make sure you work on the correct side joints and the correct side LEFT/RIGHT

    Step 3: Bend and Straighten the resident's ARM holding the ELBOW, towards the shoulder and straighten it back towards the mattress. This process is called FLEXION/EXTENSION. Repeat this process THREE TIMES.

    Step 4: Move the WRIST by bending it DOWN and BACK UP . This process is called FLEXION/HYPEREXTENSION. Repeat the process THREE TIMES

    Step 5: Ensure you maintain face contact with the patient so you can see if he/she is in pain or discomfort

Step 6: Close your skill by ensuring the resident is fine and is not in need of anything else before leaving the room. Always offer the patient water, cold or room temperature before you leave the resident's room

Step 7: Remember to lower the bed to a case level if you had raised it up to the skill.

Finish with your closing statement

Step 8: Ensure you wash your hands physically or verbally

Chapter 5

e

Passive range of motion
(ROM) exercises to one hip, knee and ankle

This skill takes 4-5 minutes to be completed.

There are no supplies for this skill.

T

his skill provide range of motion exercise to the resident knee and hip by FLEXING/EXTENDING them. Next you are going to DORSIFLEXION/PLANTAR and end the exercise by doing FLEXION the ANKLE Repeat this process THREE TIMES Make sure you exercise the right joints

Step 1 : Begin with your opening statement

Step 2: Raise the resident's hip and knee towards the torso and back towards the mattress. This is called FLEXION/EXTENSION. Repeat this process THREE TIMES, slowly and gently.

Step 3: Make sure you hold the resident's extremity to prevent heel friction against the mattress while doing the exercise

Step 4: Raise resident's foot up toward head and point downwards towards the mattress. This is called DORSIFLEXION/PLANTAR FLEXION. Do this THREE TIMES slowly and gently.

Step 5: Support resident's leg during care.

Step 6: Maintain eye contact, ensure communication by asking for patient's preferences and needs.

Step 7: Close your skill by ensuring the resident is fine and is not in need of anything else before leaving the room. Always offer the patient water cold/room temperature.

Step 8: Remember to lower bed , before you leave the room depending on whether you raised or not during the skill.

Finish your skill by the closing statement

Step 9: Ensure you wash your hands physically or verbally

e

Change Position

The time required for this skill is 8-11 minutes.

Supplies: 4 - One towel/barrier and three pillows.

T

his skill requires that you change the position of a patient who is lying on his/her back to a side lying position. The patient requires support to remain on this side, in order to make sure they do not get bedsores.

Begin with your opening statement and perform the necessary procedures. Then follow the steps listed below

> **Step 1:** Help your patient come closer to you before turning them to a side lying position to ensure they remain in the middle of the bed (checkpoint) after turning them to a side lying position

> **Step 2**: Help your patient fold their arms and bend their knees before turning them, you cannot turn the patient unless the knees are bent.

> **Step 3:** Place the first pillow/padding against patient's back and tuck it in securely underneath the patient's back. This is to make sure that the patient does not roll back and that the patient remains on a side lying position with upper knee bent in front of lower leg

> **Step 4:** Place the second pillow/padding between patient's legs so that bony prominences of the knees and ankles are separated

Step 5: Place the third pillow/padding positioned under the resident's upper arm, supporting both the shoulder and the arm

Step 6: Leave the resident positioned on his/her side without lying on the shoulder, arm and hand (checkpoint)

Step 7: Because the patient has moved. ensure the head is positioned in the middle of the pillow, and the neck and chin are both on the pillow (checkpoint)

Step 8: Maintain eye contact, ensure communication by asking for patient's preferences and needs.

Step 9. :Then close your skill as usual

Step 10: Wash your hands physically or verbally

Chapter 7

e

Assist resident with Bedpan

The time required for this skill is 8-11 minutes.

Supplies: 7 - one towel/barrier, bedpan, toilet paper, chuck, wipes/warm washcloth, 2 set of gloves.

T

he skill is performed on a person dressed in a hospital gown and pretending not to be wearing underpants. Checkpoints for this skill are: Make sure you wear gloves to place the chuck underneath the resident who is positioned on one side . Lower the head of the bed to remove the chuck and have your resident raise their hips to remove the chuck. Raise the head of the bed before the resident uses the bedpan, Make sure the bedpan is positioned according to the form and shape to allow collection. Offer assistance to the resident before you leave the room Give the resident the call light before you leave the room to them them privacy. Change gloves when you return to the room to remove the bedpan and chuck. Offer the resident wipes after they use the bedpan

Step 1 : Begin with your opening statement

Step 2: Ms Suzie i understand you want to use the Bedpan is that correct?

Step 3: Ask the resident if you can use their overbid table and let them know you will return it back to them after you complete the skill.

Step 4: Put the towel barrier on the patient's table

Step 5: Put all 6 remaining supplies on the protected over-bed table: bedpan, wipes, toilet paper, chuck, and two sets of hand gloves

Step 6: Put on the first set of gloves and then ask the patient to turn to the side lying position

Step 7: Place protective pad (chuck) on the bed over bottom sheet underneath patient's buttock/upper thigh area.

Step 8: Have your resident turns to one side to place the Bedpan underneath the resident buttocks and make sure the bedpan is positioned to allow collection

Step 9: Raise the head of bed so that the patient can be sitting on their buttocks to use the bathroom. It is more comfortable to use the bathroom sitting than laying on your back

Step 10: Give the patient toilet paper and offer assistance to the patient before leaving the room to give them privacy

Step 11: Place the call light within reach so that the resident can call you when they need help or when they are done using the bathroom

Step 12: Take off the first set of gloves and dispose them when exiting the room and then step outside to give the patient privacy

Step 13: Return to the room once the patient announces that he/she is done.

Step 14: Put on the second pair of gloves as soon you enter the resident's room and then offer the patient wipes or warm wash clothes to wipe their hands

Step 15: Lower the head of the bed so that the resident is back on a lying position. This makes it easy to remove the bedpan

Step 16: Once the resident is back to a lying position. Ask the patient raise buttock/hips so you can remove the bedpan and chuck at the same time underneath the resident. Make sure the chuck covers the bedpan

Step 17: Grab the call light with a napkin and place it within the resident's reach and lower the bed before you walk away from the resident to dispose and clean the contents of the bedpan.

Step 18: pour the contents of the bedpan in the commode/toilet.

Step 19. Rinse the bedpan and pour the dirty water in the toilet/commode three times, sanitize the bedpan and dry the bedpan completely.

Step 20: Grab a two napkins –hold the bedpan with one napkin, use the other napkin to place toilet paper and wipes in the bedpan and put everything in the third drawer

Step 21: Remove the barrier off the table and place it in a dirty hamper

Step 22: Take off your gloves

Step 23: Place the resident's over-bed table next to her with fresh water

Step 24: Tidy up the bed linen and empty trash

Step 25: Leave the patient positioned safely in the middle of the bed

Step 26: Maintain eye contact, ensure communication by asking for patient's preferences and needs.

Step 27: Close your skill by ensuring the resident is fine and is not in need of anything else before leaving the room. Always offer the patient fresh water

Step 28: Check to make sure the bed is lowered, the call light is within the resident's reach.

Step 29: Finish your skill with your closing statement.

Step 30: Ensure you wash your hands physically or verbally

Chapter 8

e

Measure and record
a resident's radial pulse

The time required for this skill is 4-5 minute.

Supplies: Clock with a second hand to count the seconds and a recording sheet.

I

t is important to note that the normal resting heart rate is 60-100 BPM for an adult. This skill demands that you take the patient's radial pulse. Which is located on lateral of the wrist. The pulse will be counted for one full minute. A measurement form is supplied to record the pulse rate. The examiner will hold the resident's one hand, while the student holds the other hand to ensure accuracy. The student is expected to have the same reading as the examiner or allow to be at the most FOUR POINTS apart in order to pass this skill

Step 1: Begin with an opening statement, ensure privacy and wash your hands

Step 2: Rub your hand together to make sure they are nice and warm before you touch the resident

Step 3: Support patient's arm such that it won't hang down while taking the pulse, and ask the resident to be still and quite

Step 4: Ensure that the patient is relaxed for the accurate resting heart beat

Step 5: Straighten the patient's elbow and face the inside of the wrist upward

Step 6: Position the index and middle fingers of your dominant hand together on wrist of the resident below the thumb

Step 7: Count one full minute

Step 8: Avoid using your thumb when taking pulse

4 beats per minutes of the examiner/nurse's measurement

Step 9: Maintain eye contact, ensure communication by asking for patient's preferences and needs. Then close your skill as usual

Step 10: Record your count on the measurement sheet provided after you wash your hands.. Bare in mind your score should be within +/- 4 to pass the skill

Step 11: Always ask resident if they are okay through the skill, to ensure maximum comfort and minimum discomfort.

Step 12: Close your skill, by making going through your closing statement.

Step 13: Make sure to wash hands physically if the first of the exam or verbally by pretending if this is the second or third skill

Step 14: Lastly do not forget to lower bed place the Call light next to the patient's hand

Chapter 9

e

Measure and record
a resident's respirations

The time required for this skill is 4-5 minutes.

Supplies: A clock with a second to count in seconds

I

t should be noted that the normal respiratory rate for a healthy adult is
12-20. Normal respiration consists of deep even breaths during which the
rib cage fully contracts and relaxes. One respiration consists of one
complete rise and fall of the chest or the inhalation and exhalation of air.
This skill demands that you count patient's respirations for ONE FULL
minute. The skill is done by the examiner and the student on another
student who is role playing the resident's role A measurement form is
also provided for record purposes.

   Step 1: Begin with your opening statement

   Step 2: Stand/sit next to the patient, hold their arm and watch their
chest for rising and falling

   Step 3: Do not give instructions to the patient not to breathe. Ensure
the patient is in a relaxed position for accuracy

   Step 4: The examiner and the student are going to count the number of
the resident's chest rise and fall within 1 minute.

Step 5: Record the count result on the measurement sheet provided. You are allowed to be within +/- 2 breaths per minute of the examiner/nurse's measurement

Step 6: Maintain eye contact, ensure communication by asking for patient's preferences and needs.

Step 7: Always ask resident if they are okay through the skill, to ensure maximum comfort and minimum discomfort.

Step 8: Finish the skill by going through the closing statement .

Step 9: Make sure to wash hands physically if the first of the exam or verbally by pretending if this is the second or third skill

Step 10: Lastly do not forget to lower bed, place the Call light next to the patient's hand

Chapter 10

e

Change Bed Linen while
the Resident remains in Bed

You are required to perform this skill within 12-15minutes.

Supplies: 5 - 1 towel/barrier, top sheet, bottom sheet, 1 pillow case and 1 blanket.

T

his skill tests you on changing the resident's bed linen while resident stays in the bed. Checkpoints : Keep resident in the middle of the bed throughout the skill. Make sure the resident's body does not touch the uncovered mattress, Make sure the resident remains on the bottom sheet through the skill. Make sure you avoid pulling the sheet in a way that it causes friction or skin shearing. Make sure the bottom sheets is free of creases or folds. Tuck the top sheet under the resident's foot of mattress, but make sure its loose enough to avoid pressure on the toes and allow them to move freely. Make sure the resident's head remains on the pillow except when changing the pillow case

Step 1: Begin with the opening statement-

Step 2: Politely request to use the over bed table of your patient to put all supplies for the skill

Step 3: Put the barrier and the four remaining supplies on the table

Step 4: Replace the patient's top sheet by the temporary blanket, and asking the resident to hold the corners of the blanket while you gently remove the soiled sheet away from the patient,

Step 5: Put the soiled sheet in the dirty hamper

Step 6: Untuck all corners of the bottom sheet

Step 7: Help the patient move towards you to prepare them to turn to the side lying position,

Step 8: Roll in the soiled linen, and replace it with the clean linen halfway through the bed, While making sure the resident's body remains on the linen. Make sure the resident's body is turned away from the side you are working on.

Step 9: Once you have securely tucked in the clean sheet one side.

Step 10: Go around to other side of the bed and help the patient move close towards you gently without creating friction to avoid the risk of skin shearing on their delicate skin

Step 11 : Help your resident to turn on a side lying position.

Step 12: Pull out the remaining soiled linen and pull out the clean linen to make sure your resident remains on the sheet throughout the skill and not exposed to the uncovered mattress

Step13: Put the soiled linen in the dirt hamper

Step 14: Secure the clean bottom sheet to mattress, making sure it is fitted on all four corners, and tucked at the head of the bed and at the bottom of the mattress, and all sides, and it does not have creases to avoid bedsores

Step 15: Tuck the top sheet underneath the resident's foot of mattress leaving sheet placed loosely, avoiding pressure against toes and allowing for foot movement

Step 16: Ask the resident to lift up their head so that you can remove the soiled pillow and change the pillow case away from the resident. Place the soiled pillow case in dirty hamper once you take it off

Step 17: Fold the pillow and insert into the clean pillow case and place the clean pillow underneath the resident

Step 18: Leave top sheet placed on top of resident to cover body up to shoulder level, without tucking in along sides

Step 19: Maintain eye contact, ensure communication by asking for patient's preferences and needs. T

Step 20: Finish your skill by going through closing statement

Step 21: Make sure to wash hands physically if the first of the exam or verbally by pretending if this is the second or third skill

Chapter 11

e

Transfer the resident from
the bed into a wheelchair using a pivot technique and a transfer/gait belt

The time required for this skill is 8-11 minutes.

Supplies: 2 - Wheelchair and gait, non-skid socks/shoes

T

his skill tests you on transferring a patient who is lying in bed into a wheelchair. using the pivot technique The checkpoints are: Assist and support the resident to a sitting position on the side of the bed without pulling the resident arms or hands. Make sure your resident has shoes on before their feet touch the floor, make sure you gait belt is on the resident's waist over their clothing before they stand, make sure sure the resident is not dizzy after they stand and before you transfer them using a pivot technique into the wheelchair. Make sure resident does not take a step to reach wheelchair, use proper body mechanics . This skill is done by a person.

Step 1: Begin with the opening statement

Step 2: Place wheelchair close to the bed. without blocking the resident when they stand

Step 3 : Assist and support the resident into a sitting position without pulling on arms or hands

Step 4: Position the resident to sit on the side of the bed

Step 5: Place the resident's shoes or nonskid footwear on the patient before you make the patient stand for transfer

Step 6: Make sure that the wheelchair footrests are not in the way before you make the patient stand for transfer (e.g., lift, swing, or remove)

Step 7: Place the transfer/gait securely around the patient's waist and over the clothing in such a way that only flat fingers fit under the belt. Ensure that the belt does not affect the skin or skin folds

Step 8 : Position the resident's feet flat on the floor before you assist them to stand on their feet

Step 9: Position the wheelchair ready for transfer by positioning the front interior wheel close to the bed so the you can just transfer the resident with a pivot technique the resident taking a step to reach the wheelchair

Step 10 : Lock the wheelchair before transfer

Step 11: Position yourself in front of the resident supporting him by holding the transfer/gait belt at sides or around the back all through the transfer

Step 12 : Assist your resident to stand by holding on to the gait belt around their waist. Ask your resident if they are okay or DIZZY

Step 13 : Give your resident a signal when you are ready to transfer them to the wheelchair

Step 14: Support either one or both of the patient's legs throughout transfer while helping the resident to turn, sit

Step 15: Use your body mechanics while helping the patient to transfer into the wheelchair and using a PIVOT TECHNIQUE

Step 16: Ensure the patient's body is properly aligned, hips against back of the seat, and feet is on footrests

Step 17: After the transfer is complete, remove the transfer/gait belt carefully without causing harm to the patient

Step 18: Maintain eye contact, ensure communication by asking for patient's preferences and needs.

Step 19: Close your skill, by making sure the resident is okay and does need anything else before leaving the room.

Step 20: Make sure to wash hands Physically if this is the first of the exam or Verbally by pretending if this is the second or third skill

Step 21: Lastly do not forget to lower bed place the Call light next to the patient's hand

Chapter 12

e

Ambulate the resident using a Transfer/Gait Belt

This skill lasts for 4-5 minutes.

Supplies: 2 - Gait belt, non-skid socks or shoes

T

he skill tests you on assisting a resident with standing and walking. You will need to use a transfer gait belt to help the resident stand and walk 10 steps. The checkpoints for the skill are: Make sure you put the transfer gait on the resident, Make you ask the patient if they are dizzy or not upon standing. Make sure you walk on the WEAK SIDE of the patient slightly behind them.

Step 1: Begin with the opening statement

Step 2: Place the transfer/gait belt securely around the patient's waist and on top of their clothing in such a   way that flat fingers fit under the belt.

Step 3 : Make sure the transfer gait belt does not attach to the skin or skin folds

Step 4 : Give your resident a signal before making stand

Step 5: Help the patient to his/her feet while holding the transfer/gait belt and ask them "Are you okay are you DIZZY ?

Step 6: Support your resident with your arm around their back while you are walking them

Step 7 :Walk your resident 10 steps by positioning yourself slightly behind them on their WEAK SIDE,

Step 8: Ask the resident how they feel during ambulation

Step 9: When you finish walking resident, make sure the resident's back of the leg touches against the seat before you help them to seat. Remember always to use your body mechanics

Step 10: Help the patient onto the seat and take away transfer/gait belt

Step 11: Ensure the patient is seated appropriately with their back on the chair and leg on the footrest

Step 12: Maintain eye contact, ensure communication by asking for patient's preferences and needs.

Step 13: Finish your skill by going through closing statement

Step 14: Make sure to wash hands physically if the first of the exam or verbally by pretending if this is the second or third skill

Chapter 13

e

Dress Resident who has a weak arm

Time required to complete the skill: 12-15 minutes.

Supplies: 5 - 1 Towel/Barrier 2 sets of pants, 2 long sleeve button-front shirts, a pair of socks.

T

his skill tests you on dressing a resident who has weak side. eg a Stroke resident is paralyzed on one side. The risen is going to be lying in bed and wearing a hospital gown. Checkpoints : Pick two outfits for the resident and let them choose the outfit they want to wear. Undress the resident from the hospital gown. Dress a resident into a long-sleeved button-front shirt, pants, and socks .The patient cannot dress him/herself because of a weak arm. A mannequin will be our resident. Here is the acronym to remember: USDW: Undress from strong and dress from weak side: Meaning; undress from Strong side because the resident can bend their arm to help you, and Dress from the First because they cannot bend their arm

Step :1 Begin with the opening statement-

Step :2: Before you can do anything you need to place a towel/barrier on the over bed table for all your supplies

Step 3: Pick two outfits from the supply closet, give the resident a choice to pick whichever outfit they like.

Step 4: Place the outfit they chose on the over bed table that is covered by the barrier

Step 5 : Place the blanket over the resident, and pull their top sheet down

Step 6: Untyre and unbutton the resident's hospital gown by starting on the STRONG SIDE FIRST, support the affected arm while undressing resident

Step 7: Put the soiled gown in the dirty hamper

Step 8: Dressing the resident with the socks first, gather the socks first before you apply them on the resident to make sure you avoid skin shearing

Step 9: Put on the resident's pants, bunch up the pants to allow easy access up to the waistline

Step 10 :Once you get to the waistline. Raise the head of the bed up and allow your resident to sit up if possible. Its easier to have your resident lean forward than to roll them to a side lying position incase they land on their weak arm.

Step 11: Dressing the resident, from the WEAK SIDE first, gather the shirt sleeve up for easy access and slide up the weak arm FIRST

Step 12 : Tuck in the rest of the shirt behind the resident ,so that you can just pull it when you get to the other side.

Step 13: Go to the other side of the resident pull the tucked shirt gently and gather up the sleeve again. Ask your resident to bend their strong Arm and slide the shirt in. Make sure you don not over extend the arm or apply force to to the resident's extremities.

Step 14: Make sure the shirt is tucked in neatly and securely with all the shirt buttons, buttoned up

Step 15: Place all the soiled garments and towels in a dirty hamper

Step 16: Ensure the resident is always positioned in the safely in the middle of the bed

Step 17: Maintain eye contact, ensure communication by asking for patient's preferences and needs.

Step 18: Finish your skill by going through the closing statement

Step 19: Make sure to wash hands physically if this is the first skill of the exam or verbally by pretending if this is the second or third skill

Step 20: Lastly do not forget to lower bed place the Call light next to the patient's hand

Chapter 14

e

Empty resident's urinary drainage bag contents, and measure and record urine output on an Intake and Output (I&O) form.

The Time required for this skill is 8-11 Minutes.

Supplies: 5 - chuck/barrier graduate, 1 pair of gloves, a tissue and alcohol pads.

T

his skill involves emptying the resident's urinary drainage bag into a graduate container and measuring and record the amount and the time of the urine. An Intake and Output (I&O) Form will be provided by the examiner to record the measurement. For the purpose of the exam, urine is going to be drained in the GRADUATE and recorded in Centiliters (CC) along with the precise time. The skill can be done to a person/mannequin

Step 1: Begin with the opening statement-

Step 2: Place a chuck as barrier on the floor before you can put any supplies

Step 3: Pull out your graduate from the bottom last drawer and place it along with your other supplies on top of the barrier on the floor.

Step 4: Put on your gloves

Step 5: Raise the resident's bed to make sure the graduate does not touch the drainage bag

Step 6: Check catheter tubing under the resident's blanket to make sure its not kinked.

Step 7: Position the graduate or bedpan on the floor and pour out the full contents of the drainage bag into the bedpan or graduate.

Step 8 ;Ensure this is done without contaminating the drainage tube by touching container for example. (e.g. clamp and tuck drain into pocket) after pouring out the contents of the drainage bag

Step 9 : Use your alcohol pad to clean up the pout of drainage bag before tucking it back in and dispose the trash in a trash bin

Step 10: Slide the chuck/graduate away from the bed and take the tissue paper to lower the bed to a safe level before walking away from the resident to dispose off the urine

Step 11: Position the graduate on a flat surface with barrier/chuck to take measurement by reading the graduate at eye level. YOU ARE ALLOWED TO BE WITHIN +/- 50 ML OF EXAMINER'S measurement

Step 12 : Pour contents in the commode/toilet, dispose of the chuck in the trash bin if disposable. or soiled the hamper if reusable

Step 13: Rinse the GRADUATE 3 Times, while pouring every rinse in the commode/toilet dry the GRADUATE, disinfect and dry it completely.

Step 14 : Grab two napkins: One to hold the graduate the second one to open the resident's drawer to place back her graduate in the bottom last drawer

Step 15: Remove gloves before you commence documentation.

Step 16: Document the OUTPUT **WITH CLEAN HANDS**

Step 17: Make sure the urine bag is placed at a position lower than the bladder all through the care, and ensure the bag is not hanging on the side rail only BED FRAME

Step 18: Always ask resident if they are okay through the skill, to ensure maximum comfort and minimum discomfort.

Step 19: Finish your skill, by going through the closing statement

Step 20: Make sure to wash hands physically if the first of the exam or verbally by pretending if this is the second or third skill

Step 21: Lastly do not forget to lower bed place the Call light next to the patient's hand

Chapter 15

e

Feed a resident who is sitting in a chair

The Time required for this skill is 8-11 Minutes.

Supplies: 8 - Tray, Bib/towel wipes/wet wash cloth, spoon, Folk, knife, snack (jello/pudding).

T

his skill you are being tested on feeding a resident a snack and fluid intake to a resident who unable to feed him/herself. The resident is sitting in a chair in an improper pose for feeding. A Food and Fluid Intake Form is provided to record the resident's estimated food and fluid intake. The role of the resident is played by a person. You also want to engage the resident in a conversation while eating to encourage more intake. It is important to sit facing the resident while feeding them.

Step 1 : Begin with the opening statement-

Step 2: The Snack will be placed on the table for the resident by the examiner on a napkin

Step 3: Bring the patient to an upright sitting position before feeding

Step 4: Use a damp washcloth, paper, towel or hand wipe to wash patient's hands before feeding, and dispose in trash bin

Step 5 : Put the barrier around the resident's neck and clothing to protect their clothing

Step 6 : Sit facing the resident so you can be at eye level and able to observe any difficulty with chewing or swallowing

Step 7 : Open all the food/snack container for the patient to see, and ask them which food choice do they want to start with

Step 8: Offer the resident water before feeding them to moisten their mouth

Step 9 : Use the spoon to feed the resident to avoid poking them with a sharp object

Step 10 : Feed the resident 3/4 of the spoon and allow them to swallow

Step 11 : Give patient fluid to drink after every 2-3 bites of spoon feeding through the feeding.

Step 12: Wait for the patient to swallow before offering the next bite

Step 13: Create conversation with the patient during meal to encourage the patient to eat more

Step 14: Dispose all of the resident's unfinished food and the water cup in a trash bin

Step 15 : Remove the resident bib/barrier after the resident is done eating, and place the garment in the soiled linen hamper or trash bin if you used disposable bib

Step 16 : Leave the resident's table clean and dry the patient's mouth when care has been completed

Step 17 : Finish your skill by going through the closing statement and wash your hands

Step 18: Record the resident's food and fluid intake amount on the measurement form provided. You should be WITHIN 25% OF THE EXAMINER'S MEASUREMENT

Step 19: Always ask resident if they are okay through the skill, to ensure maximum comfort and minimum discomfort.

the room.

Step 20: Make sure to wash hands physically if the first of the exam or verbally by pretending if this is the second or third skill

Step 21: Lastly do not forget to lower bed place the Call light next to the patient's hand

Chapter 16

e

Provide catheter care to a female resident who has an indwelling urinary catheter

The Time required for this skill is 12-15 Minutes.

Supplies: 13 - 1 towel/Barrier, 1 Chuck, 4 washcloths, 2 Big Towels, 2 pairs of gloves, 1 blanket, 1 Basin, and Soap.

T

his skill you are going to be tested on cleaning a female patient with soap and water who has indwelling Urinary Cather as well cleaning the perennial area Because this skill is more invasive the mannequin is used. Because the test is more for the Catheter care you are not required to clean the rectal area. ONLY THE FRONT PART.

Step 1 : Begin with the opening statement

Step 2: Place the barrier on the table

Step 3: Place all the supplies on the table that is covered by the barrier

Step 4: Put on gloves

Step 5: You want to prepare your patient before you fetch the water, so that the water is not cold by the time you clean the patient

Step 6 :Help the resident to turn to a side lying position so that you can the chuck underneath the resident's buttons to make sure you get the bottom sheet wet.

Step 7: Place the blanket over the patient and pull their top sheet down to protect it from the getting wet

Step 8: Once you have prepared the patient for catheter care, remove the gloves and fetch the water, with bare hands so that you can test the temperature of the water with your bare hands before you take the water to the resident to test it too to make are its lukewarm

Step 9: Have the resident test the water temperature before you can put it on the table along with the rest of the supplies

Step 10: Put on the second pair of gloves

Step 11 : Place all your 4 wash clothes in the water basin

Step 12: Take the first wash cloth out of the water and fold it into 4 pieces and apply soap to all the 4 corners

Step 13 : Start by checking the catheter tubing to make sure its not kinked or tangled up

Step 14: Wash the catheter tubing about 3-4 inches away from the body with soapy cloth and changing positions on the wash cloth

Step 15 : Place the soiled washcloth in the dirty hamper

Step 16 : out of the water and apply soap to Start by taking the first washcloth to wash the catheter, ensure that catheter is held near meatus to avoid pulling when handling.

Step 17: Wash away from body and down the catheter at least 3-4 inches with soapy washcloth

Step 18: Take the second washcloth and rinse off the catheter and dispose the wet wash cloth in the dirty hamper

Step 19: Take the big towel and pat dry the resident

Step 20 : Fold the third washcloth and apply soap to the all the four corners away from the basin

Step 21 : Clean the Meatus first, front to back, then labia one and two , skin fold and pubic bone with soap, going from front to back. Dispose the soiled wash cloth in the dirty hamper

Step 22: Take the fourth washcloth and rinse the inside the meatus, labia one and two, skin fold and then pubic bone front to back Dispose the soiled wash cloth in the dirty hamper

Step 23: Pat dry the perineal area front to back

Step 24: Keep tubing free from kinks or obstruction. Also keep tubing and urinary drainage bag off the ground

Step 25: Make sure the urinary drainage bag in a position lower than bladder all the time

Step 26: Rinse, disinfect the basin and dry. Place soiled linens in hampers, dispose trash and leave over bed table with a pitcher of fresh water and a cup

Step 27: Always maintain patient in a safe distance from the bed's edge

Step 28: Always ask resident if they are okay through the skill, to ensure maximum comfort and minimum discomfort.

Step 29: Finish your skill, by going through the closing statement

Step 30: Make sure to wash hands physically if the first of the exam or verbally by pretending if this is the second or third skill

Step 31: Lastly do not forget to lower bed place the Call light next to the patient's hand

Chapter 17

e

Provide Foot care to
patient who is sitting

The to complete the skill: 12-15 Minutes.

Supplies: 7 - Chuck/barrier, 1 big towel, basin, 1washcloth, soap, lotion, 1 pair of gloves.

T

his skill You are going to provide foot care to a resident who is sitting in a chair. That means you are going to be tested on washing only 1 resident's foot. You are going to have to wash a resident's foot with soap and rise it off . Once you complete washing the foot, you have to replace a resident sock and shoe back on.   patient's role is played by another student

Step 1 : Begin with the opening statement

Step 2: Place the barrier(chuck) on the floor

Step 3: Place all your supplies on the chuck

Step 4: Get lukewarm water and have the resident, test the water before you can use on the resident

Step 5: Position a basin that is filled with warm water on a protective barrier on the floor in preparation for foot care

Step 6: Put on gloves

Step 7: Remove the 1 shoe, and sock from the resident and soak the foot for about 10 minutes

Step 8: Remove the foot from the water basin and wash it with soapy wash cloth on top of the folded towel NOT INSIDE THE BASIN WITH WATER

Step 9: Place the resident's foot back in the basin to rinse it without any wash cloth. Ensure the top and bottom of foot is washed. Also wash the toes and in between toes

Step 10: Change position of the towel before placing wet foot back on the towel

Step 11 : Pat dry the resident's foot especially between the toes.

Step 12: Change position again on the towel and proceed to Put lotion on your hands and rub them together to make the lotion is warm

Step 13: Apply the warm lotion over the foot except in between the toes and remove excess from toes after applying

Step 14: Put on the sock on the foot and the shoe. Secure every fastener on the shoe

Step 15: Do not, at any point, put the patient's barefoot directly on the floor

Step 16: Pour the dirty water in the toilet and Rinse, the basin 3 times, disinfect and dry basin.

Step 17: Use the barrier to hold the basin and another barrier to open the resident storage place and put the supplies away.

Step 18: Remove the chuck from the floor and Place soiled linen in hamper, and remove your gloves

Step 19 : Empty the trash

Step 20: Leave the resident with a pitcher of fresh water and a cup on the over bed table

Step 21: Always ask resident if they are okay through the skill, to ensure maximum comfort and minimum discomfort.

Step 22: Finish your skill, by going through the closing statement

Step 23: Make sure to wash hands physically if the first of the exam or verbally by pretending if this is the second or third skill

Step 24: Lastly do not forget to lower bed place the Call light next to the patient's hand

e

Provide mouth care to
a resident who has a denture

The time required to complete the skill: 12 - 15 Minutes.

Supplies:12 - 1 towel/barrier, Dentures, toothpaste, Denture brush, emesis basin, 2 washcloths- 1 -barrier for the sink, 2nd wash cloth to pat dry the resident, bib/towel, cup of water, 2 pairs of gloves, toothette

T

he skill tests you on cleaning the resident's dentures and mouth. The checkpoints for this skills are: Preparing the sink to clean the denture by lining the sink with a wash cloth or filling the sink with water. Using lukewarm water to clean the dentures with denture toothbrush and toothpaste while wearing gloves. After cleaning dentures you have to change gloves, use emesis basin, tootheete, cup of water to clean the resident's gums while protecting the resident's clothing with a bib/towel. Rinsing the resident's mouth after brushing and pat drying resident between brushing and the rinsing. Lastly finishing the skill by cleaning the emesis basin and dissecting it and disposing all the soiled linen in the dirty hamper

Step 1 : Begin with the opening statement-

Step 2: Place the barrier on the table

Step 3: Place all the supplies on the table that is covered by the barrier

Step 4: Take the first wash cloth from your supplies on the table and place in the sink where are going to clean the denture. You can also feel the sink with water to protect the dentures

Step 5: Put on your gloves

Step 6: Apply toothpaste on the denture toothbrush, place the denture toothbrush in the emesis basin, take the dentures in their case, and bring them to the sink area

Step 7: Place the denture toothbrush, and the emesis basin on a barrier around the sink area.

Step 8: Remove the dentures out of the denture cup, rinse the denture cup three times and fill it up with cool water, then place it on a barrier around the sink

Step 9: Run cool /tepid water to brush all surfaces of the dentures thoroughly with toothpaste

Step 10 : Pick out any food substances stuck between dentures with the pick on the other side of the denture brush if you need to.

Step 11 : Rinse the dentures and remove the toothpaste with cool running water, not water inside the sink

Step 12: Place clean dentures in clean cool water in the denture cup

Step 13 : Remove the barrier out of the sink and place it in the soiled hamper

Step 14: Bring back the clean dentures in a protected cup and place them by resident's bedside table

Step 15 : Bring the denture toothbrush in the emesis basin and place them on the table with other supplies

Step 16: Change your gloves and place a bib on your resident to prepare for mouth care using a toothette and toothpaste

Step 17: Offer your resident a sip of water to moisten the mouth

Step 18: Gently swipe the resident upper and lower gums using a toothettee with toothpaste

Step 19: Provide the resident the emesis basin to spit after every brush to spit in

Step 20: Pat dry the resident

Step 21: Offer the resident water to rinse their mouth three times

Step 22 : Pat dry the resident

Step 23: Remove the bib/towel of the patient chest once you finish cleaning their mouth and place it in the soiled linen hamper

Step 24: Dispose of the cup, toothette in the trash bin

Step 25 : Take the emesis to the sink and pour out the spit in the sink and rinse, the emesis basin three times, disinfect and dry it.

Step 26: Hold the emesis basin with the barrier and hold another barrier with the other hand to open the resident storage. Place all the supplies from the table inside.

Step 27: Place the soiled linen in the dirty hamper

Step 28: Empty the trash bin and remove your gloves

Step 29: Leave the resident's over bed table with Pitcher of fresh water and a cup

Step 30: Always ask resident if they are okay through the skill, to ensure maximum comfort and minimum discomfort.

Step 31: Finish the skill by going through the closing statement .

Step 32: Make sure to wash hands physically if the first of the exam or verbally by pretending if this is the second or third skill

Step 33: Lastly do not forget to lower bed place the Call light next to the patient's hand

Chapter 19

e

Provide mouth care to
a resident who has teeth

The time required to complete the skill: 12-15 Minutes.

Supplies: 8 -1 Towel/barrier, Toothbrush, toothpaste, cup of water, emesis basin, and washcloth, 1 pair of gloves, 1 bib/towel

T

his skill tests you on brushing resident's natural teeth while lying in bed because the resident is unable to brush their own teeth. The checkpoints in the skill are: Raising the head of the bed to a 60-90 degrees so that the resident is sitting in an upright position to avoid chocking. Wearing gloves, Covering the resident's clothing with a bib or towel . Moistening the mouth and toothbrush before applying the toothpaste before brushing the resident's teeth. Brushing all sides, resident's biting surfaces including the gums. Rinsing the resident's teeth and using emesis basin for a resident to spit in. Pat drying the resident in between brushing teeth. Lastly cleaning the resident's emesis basin. Storing it away and disposing the soiled linen and leaving the resident clean and in a sitting position for 90 minutes

Step 1 : Begin with the opening statement-

Step 2: Place the barrier on the table

Step 3: Place all the supplies on the table that is covered by the barrier

Step 4: Put on your gloves

Step 5: Raise the resident's head of bed to 60-90 degrees so that the resident is sitting in an upright position.

Step 6: Cover the patient's clothing with a bib/towel

Step 7: Give the resident a sip of water to moisten the mouth. Give them an emesis basin to spit

Step 8 : Pat dry the resident with a towel

Step 9: Wet toothbrush and put toothpaste on it before you brush teeth

Step 10: Gently brush biting sides three times/ 15 seconds the surfaces of the teeth, including the gum line lastly the tongue

Step 11: Place the Emesis basin underneath the resident to spit

Step 12 : Pat dry the resident

Step 13 : Rinse the resident's mouth at least three times by giving the patient a cup of water after brushing

Step 14: Hold the emesis basin beneath the resident for spitting

Step 15: Remove the bib/towel from the resident, and dispose it in the dirty hamper

Step 16: Take the emesis basin to the sink and empty pour it in the sink

Step 17 : Rinse the emesis basin, dry it and disinfect it. Use the paper towel to hold the emesis basin after cleaning and hold another paper towel to open the resident dresser drawer and store away all other supplies

Step 18: Place soiled linens in hamper, throw away used toothbrush, disposable cup, empty trash and leave the resident over bed table with a pitcher of fresh water and a cup

Step 19: Always ask resident if they are okay through the skill, to ensure maximum comfort and minimum discomfort.

Step 20: Finish your skill by going through the closing statement

Step 21: Make sure to wash hands physically if the first of the exam or verbally by pretending if this is the second or third skill

Step 22: Lastly do not forget to lower bed place the Call light next to the patient's hand

e

Provide perineal care to a female
resident who is Incontinent of urine

The time required for this skill is 17-19 Minutes.

Supplies:14 - 1 Towel/barrier 2 chucks, 2 big towels, 4 washcloths, 1 basin, 2 pair of gloves, 1perineal soap, 1 blanket.

T

his skill tests you in giving perineal care to a female patient with urine incontinence . You will first need to change/replace the soiled chuck/underpad before you begin cleaning the resident. You will also be tested on cleaning the resident perineal area front to back as well as a Anal area. You are required to change the resident's wet temporary underpaid you placed initially before beginning the skill. You will complete your skill your leaving the resident with a clean and dry underpaid. You cannot put a soiled washcloth back in the basin with clean water. Every time you finish using the soiled wash cloth you dispose it in the soiled laundry hamperFor the purpose of this skill we are going to use Chuck/Underpad interchangeably. The role of the resident will be played by a mannequin wearing a hospital gown.

Step 1 : Begin with the opening statement-

Step 2: Place the barrier on the table

Step 3: Place all the supplies on the table that is covered by the barrier

Step 4: Put on the first set of gloves

Step 5: Assist the resident to move close you before turning them to a side lying position

Step 6 : Roll in the soiled chuck and tuck it in under the resident but on top of their bottom sheet and then insert the clean chuck so that the resident remains on a clean chuck before you begin washing the resident perineal area

Step 7: Go around to other the bed to the other side of the patient and pull out the soiled tucked chuck and throw it in the trash bin. Rollout the clean chuck

Step 8: Remove the dirty gloves, make sure the call light is close to the resident if you had moved it away **Step 9** : Take the basin from the table and get lukewarm water from the tap

Step 10 : Have your resident test the water temperature of the water before you begin the skill

Step 11: Put on your second set of gloves

Step 12: Replace the top sheet with a temporary blanket so that the top sheet does not get wet and you keep the resident warm

Step 13: Place all the washcloths in the water basin

Step 14: Begin cleaning your resident with first washcloth with soap from meatus front to back, changing the position of the washcloth, labia 1 front to back change position, labia 2, front to back change position, each skin fold front to back, and pubic bone, front to back, making sure you change position of the washcloth every time

Step 15: Take the second soap free washcloth from the basin, rinse and remove all soap from patient's perineal area and dispose the soiled washcloth in the dirty hamper

Step 16: Take the big bath towel and pat dry resident's perineal area front back

Step 17: Assist your resident to turn to a side lying position to wash the buttocks and rectal area

Step 18: Take the third wash cloth and put soap on it away from the basin and wash the resident's buttocks and rectal area, dispose the wash cloth in the soiled linen hamper

Step 19 Take the forth wash cloth and rinse the buttocks and rectal area and dispose the soiled linen in the dirty linen hamper

Step 20 : Take the basin from the table pour out everything in the toilet/commode and rinse the basin three times

Step 21: Dry and disinfect the basin with tissues provided

Step 22: Grab two tissues, use 1 tissue to hold the basin and use the other tissue to open the resident's dresser drawer and store her supplies

Step 23: Place any other soiled linen left on the table in the soiled linen hamper

Step 24: Always ask resident if they are okay through the skill, to ensure maximum comfort and minimum discomfort.

Step 25: Finish the skill by going through closing statement

Step 26: Make sure to wash hands physically if the first of the exam or verbally by pretending if this is the second or third skill

Step 27: Lastly do not forget to lower bed place the Call light next to the patient's hand

Chapter 21

e

Provide resident hand and nail care

Time required to complete the skill 8-11 Minutes.

Supplies:8 - 1 Towel/barrier, basin, soap, lotion, 1 washcloth, Emery board, orange stick, and 1big towel.

T

he skill tests your knowledge on cleaning residents's one hand, and covering all the check points for this skill which are listed below. Make sure you allow the resident to test the temperature of the water first, then soaking their hand in soap free water before washing it with a wash cloth with soap away from the basin. Then dip the resident;s soapy hand back in the clean water to rinse before proceeding to using Orange stick flat edge to remove any dirty residue under the resident's nail,, Emery board to file any jagged edges of the resident's nail., and NOT cutting the resident's nail. Applying lotion to the hand at the end of the skill It important to note that you cannot cut the resident's nails incase they are diabetic.

Step 1: Begin with your opening statement

Step 2 :Place the barrier on the table

Step 3: Place all the supplies on the table that is covered by the barrier

Step 4: Remove the basin from the table and get lukewarm water for the resident

Step 5: Have the resident check the water temperature

Step 6: Soak the resident's fingers or nails into a bowl of lukewarm water for a while

Step 7: Place the washcloth in the water basin

Step 8: Fold the wash cloth into Four sections

Step 9: Remove hand from basin and place it on top of the big towel to wash

Step 10: Take the washcloth from the basin and apply soap on it wash the hand on top of the folded towel.

Step 11: Insert the resident's soapy hand back into the clean soap free water to rinse

Step 12 : Remove the reside't hand again from the basin and place it on the dry part of the towel to wipe off the water dry. focusing between the fingers,

Step 13: Use the orange wood stick to remove residue from fingernail's tips by using flat edge of orange wood stick. Clean the orange wood stick before using it on another fingernail

Step 14: Use the emery board to smooth away the jagged edges, while hand is still resting on the towel

Step 15: Fold away another section of the towel and place the resident's hand, warm the lotion by rubbing your hands together, before massaging your resident's hand with lotion

Step 16: Wipe off the excess lotion from hand and the resident's hand dry nails smooth

Step 18 : Dispose all soiled supplies in the dirty hamper

Step 19: Take the basin and pour out the water in the sink

Step 20 : Rinse, disinfect and dry the basin THREE Times.

Step 21: Grab two napkins; first one hold the basin and the second one to open the dresser and store away all the supplies

Step 22: Dispose away the, emery board, and orange wood stick.

Step 23 :trash and finally leave the over bed table with a pitcher of fresh water and a cup

Step 24: Always ask resident if they are okay through the skill, to ensure maximum comfort and minimum discomfort.

Step 25: Finish your skill by going through the closing statement .

Step 26: Make sure to wash hands physically if the first of the exam or verbally by pretending if this is the second or third skill

Chapter 22

e

Provide resident a partial
bed bath and back rub

The time required for this skill is 17-19 Minutes.

Supplies:14 - 1 Towel/barrier, 2 big towels, 5 washcloths, soap, lotion, 2 pair of gloves, clean hospital gown, blanket

T

his skill tests you on bathing a FEMALE patient who is in bed. This patient is unable to bathe him/herself, so you are going to bathe, the face WITHOUT SOAP, and the remaining half of the body with SOAP, and that includes Neck, Chest including the breath and underneath the breast using the back of your hand to lift the resident breast, One Hand, Arm, Abdomen and lastly the Back, before dressing the resident in a clean Hospital Gown. Mannequin will be used for the purpose of the test, Make sure you don't put any SOAP in the basin

Step 1: Begin with your opening statement

Step 2 : Place the barrier on the table

Step 3: Place all the supplies on the Over bed table that is covered by the barrier

Step 4: Put on your first pair of gloves

Step 5 : Replace the top sheet with a blanket to keep the resident warm during the bath and protect the top sheet from water

Step 6: Help the resident slide close to you before turning them to their side lying position to place a towel to protect the bottom sheet, untie the soiled gown while the resident back is exposed and roll it to one side

Step 7: Place the soiled gown in the dirty hamper when you finish half of their body and ready to clean the back part

Step 8 ; Take off the first set of gloves and fetch the water with the basin and make sure its luke warm and fill the basin about 2 quarts for the exam

Step 9: Bring the water to the resident first and let them test the temperature for their own comfort level

Step 10 : Put on the second pair gloves

Step 11 : Place all the Five wash cloths in the water basin

Step 12: Use the First Soap FREE washcloth, to wash the face, starting with the EYES. Hold washcloth corners and wash the eyes from inside out changing the spot on wash cloth before cleaning the second eye

Step 13: Wash the rest of the resident's face using SOAP FREE wet washcloth,

Step 14: Dry the resident's face after washing, Do not apply any lotion

Step 15: Take the Second washcloth from the water basin, and apply soap, wash the resident's neck, chest, abdomen, up to the belly button, making sure you wash underneath resident's breast while lifting with the back of your hand, finish the skill by washing only one arm and hand.

Step 16: Take the Third washcloth rinse and remove soap from patient's neck, chest, abdomen. arm and hand and dispose it in the dirty hamper when you are done

Step 17: Dry the resident's neck, chest, abdomen, and arm with the body towel

Step 18: Help patient turn to a side lying position

Step 19: Take the Fourth washcloth and apply soap, wash the resident's back from the neck to the waistline in circular motion, and dispose wash cloth in the dirty hamper - Replace water if it becomes cold/soapy

Step 20 : Take the Fifth washcloth from the basin and rinse of the soap, and dispose wash cloth in the dirt hamper

Step 21 : Pat dry the resident's back to remove any water residue from rinsing them

Step 22: Pour lotion on your hands and rub them together to warm up the lotion before applying icon their back with long gliding and circular motion, from the waistline to the shoulders and massaging the shoulders a little bit

Step 23 : Pat dry the resident of any excess lotion and dispose the soiled towel in the dirty hamper

Step 24 : Gently remove the wet and soiled towel underneath the resident and dispose it in the dirty hamper

Step 25: Put on a clean gown on patient securing gown in back

Step 26 : Remove the wet blanket of the resident and dispose it in the dirty hamper, Pull up the resident's top sheet back on

Step 27: Lower the resident's bed and place the call light within their reach

Step 28 : Take the basin and pour out the dirty water in the sink and rise the basin 3 times and disinfect it **Step 29 :** Grab two tissues, One to hold the basin and the second one to open the resident's draw to store away her supplies, e.g lotion and soap

Step 30 : Make sure all the soiled linen is placed in the dirty hamper

Step 31: Finish your skill with the closing statement .

Step 32: Make sure to wash hands physically if this is the first skill of the exam or verbally by pretending if this is the second or third skill

Step 33: Lastly do not forget to lower bed place the Call light next to the patient's hand.

www.ingramcontent.com/pod-product-compliance
Lightning Source LLC
Chambersburg PA
CBHW071234220526
45468CB00002B/843